The Meat-only Code for Starters:

Answers to your genuine questions about the carnivore diet.

(including a 5-day meat-only eating plan!)

By

William T. Walker

Disclaimer

Table of Contents

Introduction

The meat-only diet comprises completely of meat and animal products, except every other food variety. It's professed to help weight reduction, mindset issues, and glucose stability, among other medical problems. The meat-only diet is an exclusive eating regimen that just incorporates meat, fish, and other creature food sources like eggs and certain dairy items. Except for any remaining food varieties, including organic products, vegetables, vegetables, grains, nuts, and seeds.
Its supporters likewise prescribe food varieties that are low in lactose — a sugar tracked down in milk and dairy items — like margarine and hard cheeses.

The controversial notion that our ancestors as humans ate primarily meat and fish and that high-carb diets are to blame for today's high rates of the chronic disease gave rise to the carnivore diet. Another well-known low-carb eating regimen, similar to the keto and paleo eating regimens, limits but doesn't avoid carb consumption. Nevertheless, the carnivore diet holds back nothing.

The meat-only diet or eating plan avoids all food varieties except for meat, eggs, and limited quantities of low-lactose dairy items. People who follow the diet say it can help treat some health problems, but no research backs up these claims. Following the eating regimen includes wiping out all plant food varieties from your eating routine and only eating meat, fish, eggs, and modest quantities of low-lactose dairy items.

The food varieties that are allowed include; chicken, pork, sheep, turkey, organ meats, salmon, sardines, white fish, and limited quantities of weighty cream and hard cheddar. Margarine, grease, and bone marrow are additionally permitted. Advocates of the eating routine suggest eating greasy slices of meat to arrive at your everyday energy needs. The meat-only diet advocates drinking water and bone stock while avoiding drinking tea, espresso, and different beverages produced using plants.

These diet plans may not provide much direction regarding the number of calories, serving sizes, or meals or snacks to eat each day. Most supporters of the eating regimen recommend eating as frequently as you want.

Chapter 1: What is the meat-only diet and why is everybody discussing it?

The meat-only diet (likewise called a zero-carb diet) is a prevailing fashion diet in which just products from animals like meat, eggs, and dairy are consumed. The meat-only diet is related to pseudoscientific wellbeing claims. Such an eating regimen can prompt a lack of nutrients and dietary fiber and cause an increase in the danger of succumbing to illnesses. The lion diet is a profoundly exclusive type of meat-only diet where just meat is eaten.

The German author Bernard Moncriff, who wrote The Philosophy of the Stomach in 1856, is credited with inventing the concept of a meat-only diet and he endured a year living on just meat and milk. During the 1870s, Italian doctor Arnaldo Cantani endorsed his diabetic patients with a selective meat-based diet. During the 1880s, James H. Salisbury upheld a meat diet comprising 2 to 4 pounds of lean flesh and 3 to 5 pints of high-temperature water day to day for 1 to 3 months.

It became known as the meat and temp water diet, or Salisbury diet

A meat-only eating plan or diet alludes to the eating of animal-based food sources. Individuals who follow a meat-only dietary program eat solely just meat and other flesh-based food varieties. The meat-only diet comprises solely flesh-based food varieties, like meat, fish, eggs, and low-lactose dairy. An individual following the eating routine may likewise utilize honey, salt, pepper, and zero-carb flavors.

Different food varieties — like grains, high lactose dairy, sugars, and plant-based oils — are removed from the meat-only diet. Comparable meat-weighty eating regimens, for example, ketogenic and paleolithic eating regimens, limit sugars but don't bar them by and large. Dietitians frequently allude to such eating regimens as low carb, high fat (LCHF) eating plan while, the flesh-based food varieties are referred to as the ASF diets.

The meat-only diet depends on the questionable hypothesis that human progenitors sometime in the past followed eating regimens involving lots of meats. It suggests that the human body's capability is at its best when energized by elevated degrees of protein and fat.

There are clear similarities between the paleo and meat-only diets. Both are extremely high in protein. In any case, the paleo diet permits plant-based food utilization, like organic products, veggies, and nuts. Hence, carbs cater for around 25% of the all-out energy usage, protein for around 30% of complete energy consumption, and the rest is fat.

The fundamental thought of the paleo diet is eating wild and regular food varieties, for example, natural products, veggies, meat fish, nuts, and eggs that were generally devoured during the Paleolithic period before modern cultivating techniques were created. Grains, dairy items, sugar, salt, and fast food varieties are beyond reach in the two weight control plans

Why are individuals discussing it?

The 'meat-only diet' pattern has arrived at more than a billion engagements via the online media space with some committing and gaining practical experience in the extraordinary eating regimen.

Albeit, in the same way as other weight control plans, some are addressing how safe this eating regimen is and on the off chance that there are any advantages or cons, they ought to be aware of it. The meat-only diet sees individuals centered around eating dinners that comprise a great deal of meat, including animal flesh, chicken, and pork both cooked and crude having eggs and chunks of margarine. The meat-only diet, otherwise called the zero-carb diet, is a somewhat new eating regimen pattern that has acquired notoriety lately. It includes devouring just animal products, like meat, fish, and eggs while dispensing with all plant-based food varieties from the eating regimen. The prominence of the meat-only diet can be credited to a few variables.

Right off the bat, supporters of the eating regimen guarantee that it can prompt fast weight reduction, further developed absorption, and expanded energy levels. This is because of the great protein content of animal flesh, which can assist with diminishing appetite.
The simplicity of the diet plan is another reason why the meat-only diet is so popular. Dissimilar to different weight control plans that require counting calories or following macronutrient intake, the meat eater diet just includes eating animal products, making it simple to follow and comprehend.

Besides, many individuals have revealed positive outcomes from following the meat-only diet, prompting a flood in interest and reception of the eating routine. Virtual entertainment stages, especially Instagram and Twitter, have assisted with getting the news out about the meat-only diet, with powerhouses and big names advancing the eating routine as a fast and compelling method for shedding pounds and working on by and large well-being.

Notwithstanding, it's vital to take note of the fact that the meat-only diet is a controversial eating regimen and has been condemned by numerous medical services experts and nutritionists for its expected dangers and absence of logical proof to help its cases.

Taking out all plant-based food sources from the eating routine can prompt supplement lacks, especially in fiber, nutrients, and minerals. Also, consuming a lot of animal products can raise the danger of specific medical issues, like coronary illness and particular kinds of malignant growth.

Chapter 2: Is an all-meat diet what nature expected?

Meat consumption is completely normal for humans. Anybody who says something else is uninformed or lying. We eat everything. The most bio-accessible wellspring of numerous supplements comes from eggs, organ meats, and other creature food sources. ' bio-accessible' here implies that no change step is required. For example, there is no vitamin An in plant food sources. There is beta carotene, which the vast majority can change over into vitamin A, thus I accept it is regular.

There are a few explanations behind this. The ancient man chased and ate meat, something that has gone on into current times. Certain physiological parts of people are upheld by meat, like the requirement for explicit fundamental amino acids (proteins) that are challenging to get from non-meat sources, supplements, for example, certain B nutrients that are difficult to get from non-meat sources, and our profoundly evolved cerebrums that are upheld by creature fats.

Our stomach and teeth are made to digest both meat and vegetables. Saying this doesn't imply that all meat is great or that we don't eat an excessive amount of meat.

For 95% of past human life, man ate meat he could get like fish, wild game, and little critters like bugs. Presently we eat cultivated meat normally raised unnaturally on soy and grain in feedlots and the subsequent meat may not be as nutritious for us as wild game eating their regular food sources. Furthermore, to the extent that enormous game, our predecessors endeavored to get a creature like a deer or a bison or whatever and ate for a brief time frame on the catch. Then he would need to hold on until he had the option to get one more creature for food. We can eat meat 3 feasts per day on the off chance that we can manage the cost of it and many individuals do. That might be more than our bodies were intended to consume.

For thousands of years, people have debated the natural human diet, frequently regarding the morality of eating other animals. We have a choice, while the lion does not.

Take the old Greek savant, Pythagoras for instance: " How absurd it is that flesh is made from flesh! The contention hasn't changed much for moral veggie lovers in 2,500 years. However, while people don't have the teeth or hooks of a vertebrate developed to kill and eat different creatures, that doesn't mean we aren't "assumed" to eat meat.

Our initial Homo progenitors concocted weapons and cutting apparatuses that look like sharp carnivorelike teeth. There is no great reason other than meat eating for the fossil creature bones filled with stone apparatus cut marks at fossil destinations. It also helps to explain our basic intestines, which don't look like the ones that evolved to process a lot of fibrous plant foods.

 By and by, diet masters have constructed areas of strength for a conflict between what we eat today and what our progenitors developed to eat. The term "metabolic syndrome" refers to a group of conditions that include elevated blood pressure, high blood sugar levels, obesity, and abnormal cholesterol levels.

The idea is that our diets have changed too rapidly for our genes to keep up. It makes a strong case. Just imagine what could occur assuming you put diesel in an auto instead of normal fuel. Some unacceptable fuel can unleash destruction on the framework, whether you're filling a vehicle or stuffing your face.

It makes sense, which is why Paleolithic diets continue to be so popular. There are numerous variations on the general theme, but protein- and omega-3-rich foods are consistently mentioned. Meat from a well-grass-fed cow and fish is great, and sugars ought to come from nonstarchy leafy foods. Then again, cereal grains, vegetables, dairy, potatoes, and profoundly refined and fast food varieties are out. The thought is to eat like our Stone Age progenitors — you know, spinach servings of mixed greens with avocado, pecans, diced turkey, and so forth.

Even if we were able to precisely reconstruct the nutrient composition of foods consumed by a specific hominin species in the past—which we are unable to do—the information would be useless for menu planning based on our ancestral diet.

Since our reality was truly evolving, thus, as well, was the eating routine of our predecessors. Zeroing in on a solitary point in our development would be vain. We're a work underway. Homo sapiens spread out across the land as well, and their diet likely differed from that of their lakeshore or open savanna cousins.

What was the familiar human eating routine? There is no logic to the question itself. Think about a portion of the new tracker finders who have roused Paleolithic eating regimen fans. The Tikiġaġmiut of the north Alaskan coast resided for the most part on the protein and fat of marine vertebrates and fish, though the Gwi San in Botswana's Focal Kalahari took something like 70% of their calories from carb-rich, sweet melons, and dull roots. Customary human foragers figured out how to sustain themselves from the bigger local area of life that encompassed them in a momentous assortment of territories, from close polar scopes to the jungles. Scarcely any other mammalian species can make that case, and there is little uncertainty that dietary flexibility has been critical to the achievement we've had.

Numerous paleoanthropologists today accept that the rising environment atmosphere through the Pleistocene shaped our precursors — whether their bodies their minds, or both — for the dietary adaptability that has turned into a sign of mankind. The essential thought is that our consistently impacting world winnowed out the pickier eaters among us. Nature has made us a flexible breed, which is the reason we can track down something to satisfy us on essentially the entirety of its bunch of biospheric buffet tables. It's likewise why we have had the option to change the game, progress from forager to rancher, and truly start to consume our planet.

Chapter 3: Is it safe to eat only meat?

Since it's like a ketogenic diet, and we've previously shown that meat isn't the reason for the lethal sicknesses tormenting humanity, it shows up reasonable to consider the carnivore diet ok for the vast majority — in some measure temporarily. Nevertheless, assuming that you've at any point seen the film Beverly Slopes Cop, there's one inquiry you've been kicking the bucket to pose: is all that meat going to stall out in my stomach?

The fact is that meat, like the majority of foods, is absorbed before reaching the colon in the small intestine. The possibility that meat gets affected in your digestive tract is unwarranted. It's feasible to get an internal hindrance because of illness or actual injury, yet red meat isn't something that impedes your digestive tract. Since there aren't a lot emerging, individuals who have little solid discharges will more often than not expect that waste is stalling out inside them.

However, in undeniable reality, these little developments, including those of meat-only eating regimens are just because of low admissions of fiber. Thus, the explanation for your little amount of excreta is that it doesn't have veggies in it.

A more serious worry about the meat-only diet is the danger of malignant growth. There's such a lot of proof on phytonutrients from plant food sources and how they assist with DNA security. If you're not consuming those things, nobody's entirely certain regarding what that will mean for you in the long haul. Microorganisms in the digestive tract and colon break down fiber into butyrate, a short-chain unsaturated fat. Butyrate reduces the chances of experiencing swelling in the digestive tract and possibly diminishes the danger of colon disease.

It is quite possible to think that an all-creature diet would expand your exposure to experiencing colon disease, and it's not because these animal food sources are cancer-causing in any capacity, but since you aren't likely to be eating things that assist in repressing colon malignant growth.

Having a couple of servings of red meat every week is no biggie, however, while you're eating three beef plates per day with nothing else, then that is entirely another story. You're changing the condition significantly.

Also, including fruits and vegetables in your meals has benefits for eye health, brain health, and overall longevity, and you'd be overlooking a lot of possible advantages by removing them all.

Another famous meat-only diet question;

What befalls the stomach environment?

Given the equilibrium of microscopic organisms that assist with processing your food and forestalling sickness. Certainly, those organisms should require some carbs.

A claim from famous meat-only diet practitioner says he had zero dysbiotic flora [the bad bacteria] at the end of the diet, and in his words, he claims "he had very great numbers on all the helpful microorganisms. He credits it to the meat-only diet being, if nothing else, an outrageous disposal diet that starves eager for sugar awful microbes to death".

No doubt, it would affect some of the great ones also, or perhaps we don't require a considerable lot of those. Perhaps we possibly need them on the off chance that we're eating a high-plant diet.

It's never been examined, and so for individuals to bounce right out and say that the meat-only diet is off-base and terrible for your wellbeing… indeed, we don't have the foggiest idea about that."

Does The Meat-only Diet Result in Lack of Supplements in the Body?

Casting the danger of perilous sickness aside, the meat-only diet — fairly shockingly — doesn't appear to cause many, if any, serious nutrient or mineral inadequacies. Red meat alone contains plentiful measures of iron and zinc, and fish and dairy supply vitamin D, which normally must be added to establish food varieties.

The one micronutrient that you might not necessarily get enough of is vitamin-c, which is generally very simple to get while eating plant products.

In response, meat-only supporters suggest the viewpoint that, without carbs, your body may not require a lot of vitamin-c subsequently making little levels of consumption adequate. On a fair eating routine, one of the roles of vitamin-c in the body is to produce collagen, and the amino acids you get from a huge meat consumption can take care of business without it.
To be sure, as far as we are aware, of other people following a zero-carb diet at home and abroad, none have been reported to have scurvy.

The fact is that you will get the necessary micronutrients your body needs by eating more than one variety of animal products. That implies trying out not just low-fat meats but, other food sources like; bone stock, and organ meats which have a bigger amount of micronutrients than some vegetables.

The Meat-only Diet for Sportsmen and Women

The ketogenic diet has faced a ton of intensity from pundits who say that individuals who exercise should eat carbs to supply fuel, yet science has shown that it is not only feasible to exercise on a low-carb diet, but you could perform at a top level. However, remove ALL carbs and all plant food sources and it very well may be a different story.

The short answer is that we do not yet know precisely how a long-term meat-only diet would impact muscle mass, endurance, or performance as a whole. However, many people who follow the meat-only diet claim to have made some of the best gains of their lives while following the plan.

It is important to note that, since we can live on a meat-only diet, it doesn't mean we'd fundamentally flourish with it. Assuming you're a sportsman or sportswoman, contending in running or something different that requires high results for 60-120 seconds, it would be exceptionally difficult to perform well when you're not eating any carbs.

Some individuals adjust easily to fat and their execution is not affected in any way, instead it improves, yet I figure for most people their execution will be affected. But, you'll have to give it a shot and see what happens, just like with any other diet.

On the off chance that you are a sportsperson or fitness junkie, you might want to start by adding a few vegetables to your eating regimen like broccoli, cauliflower, and kale would be appropriate. Assuming you observe that your exercises are declining, then it is advised that you add a bit of tuber or apples into the mix occasionally.

Structuring a Meat-only Eating Plan

The five-day feast plan below is an illustration of a meat-only eating plan;

Day One

Breakfast: 2 eggs, mixed in margarine, with ¼ cup cheddar on top.

Lunch: Four slices of turkey breast rolled in mozzarella cheese, as well as one cup of bone broth.

Dinner: Meatloaf.

Day Two

Breakfast: 1 cup plain yogurt and 2 hard-bubbled eggs.

Lunch: Turkey burger and 1 cup of bone stock.

Dinner: Steak of bison and sautéed shrimp on the side.

Day Three

Breakfast: Bacon and eggs.

Lunch: Soup (1 cup weighty cream and 1.5 cups bone stock with destroyed chicken thigh meat in stock).

Dinner: 6-ounce wild salmon filet, prepared or barbecued, with 1 cup of bone stock.

Day Four

Breakfast: 2 seared eggs with 3 connections of turkey hotdog.

Lunch: cotija cheese and ground chicken from one pound.

Dinner: 3 enormous meatballs (1 pound of ground hamburger, 2 eggs, ¼ cup parmesan cheddar, salt and pepper) in addition to 1 cup of bone stock.

Day Five

Breakfast: 3 cuts of turkey bacon and 2 hard-bubbled eggs.

Lunch: Wild salmon and crab burger (1 could wild salmon and 1 at any point can crabmeat blended in with 2 eggs, 2 tablespoons spread, salt and pepper) sautéed with margarine and finished off with acrid cream.

Dinner: Pizza with a chicken crust is made with one pound of ground chicken, one egg, and a round shell that is baked at 375 degrees for about 15 minutes. Take the covering out and finish off with mozzarella cheddar and turkey wiener, then, at that point, heat for an additional 15 minutes).

All meats and dairy items ought to be natural and field-raised whenever the situation allows.

Chapter 4: The Advantages and Drawdowns of a meat-only eating plan

Eating meat, meat, and more meat might seem like a bad dream to your physician, yet there are a few benefits upheld both narratively and by research.

Here are seven advantages of a meat-only eating plan;

1. You get to shed pounds easily

What happens if you eat only meat? The vast majority's most memorable response is that you'd get fat, yet that is exceptionally improbable. As with the ketogenic eating plan, not taking in carbs helps to keep your blood sugar level on the low side consistently. You don't get insulin spikes, so your body has no great explanation to store any resultant calories as a muscle-to-fat ratio. Furthermore, the limits on what you can eat make it beyond difficult to get a calorie surplus without deliberate exertion.

Ryan Munsey, a performance mentor with a degree in food science and human sustenance, has been on a ketogenic diet for a long time.

The previous fall, he explored different avenues regarding the carnivore diet for 35 days. " I wasn't attempting to get more fit," he says, "however I went from 188 to 183 pounds in the main week." Regardless of the weight reduction and the seriously confined food list, Munsey says he never felt even a little bit hungry — presumably because protein and fat are profoundly satisfying supplements. To get back into shape, Munsey found that he needed to teach himself to eat two to four pounds of meat every day.

Assuming you fall into the category of those who unconsciously munch on nuts, pretzels, or other nibble food sources, taking in many calories unknowingly, the meat-only diet can assist with putting you under control. You can't accidentally eat a hamburger or cook a steak, but it's easy to throw popcorn in your gullet. You'll start eating just as the need might arise, and taking in barely enough to keep you content. Then, you'll begin to notice the difference between physiological craving and careless eating.

2. Better Heart Well-being

The Mayo Center says your cholesterol proportion is a preferred danger indicator over all-out cholesterol or LDL. Divide your HDL score by your total cholesterol number to determine it.

A further point regarding cholesterol: even though higher LDL numbers are viewed as unsafe, the sort of LDL particles you have carried through your veins is generally significant. On the off chance that they're little and thick, they're viewed as more perilous than if they're greater and "fluffier." Thus, two individuals with a similar LDL worth could be at totally different degrees of hazard.

As per the Cooper Establishment, an effective method for figuring out what sort of LDL particles you have is to track down your proportion of fatty substances to HDL cholesterol. The lower the proportion, the less the danger. It is obvious that, if you follow this eating regimen for an exceptionally brief time frame, it will be difficult to foresee what might befall your body in the long haul, however it ought to facilitate your feelings of trepidation about the risks of meat for the cardiovascular framework.

You won't be having a heart attack after eating cow parts for five weeks. Your possibility of having one would be diminished.

3. Lower Bodily Inflammations

As per a few vegetarians, fat-rich animal food sources elevate irritation to some extent that is comparable to smoking cigarettes. The reality, notwithstanding, is that they can bring it down. A recent report in the journal Metabolism set side-by-side people who ate a high-fat, low-carb diet with those following a low-fat, high-carb diet. Calories were prohibited in the two classes, yet the high-fat eaters had lower markers of body swelling following 12 weeks. Subsequently, the specialists reasoned that high-fat eating might be more valuable to cardiovascular well-being.

The liver produces C-reactive proteins (CRP) in light of bodily inflammation, so estimating CRP levels can show how much irritation is in your framework. A degree of 10mg/L or less is typical, and 1mg/L or less is great. Munsey's CRP score post-diet was exceptionally low at 0.34.

Cutting plant food varieties from your menu can bring down body inflammations on its own. Lower irritation can mean less throbbing joints. Also, there's some proof that eating more collagen peptides, as you can obtain from bone stock, collagen, and gelatin, can further develop ligament well-being.

4. Higher Testosterone Level

Eating plans that contain high amounts of fat have been observed to help shoot up testosterone levels. As a matter of fact, a study published in the American Journal of Clinical Nutrition found that men who ate a diet high in fat and low in fiber for ten weeks had 13% more total testosterone than men who ate a diet low in fat and high in fiber.

5. Less Stomach-related Issues

We've been informed that it is so vital to eat fiber our entire lives, and have been offered everything from wheat biscuits to Metamucil to ensure we get enough. However, science may show that meat-only dieters are correct in their belief that it is more trouble than it is worth.

A recent report from the World Journal of Gastroenterology explored the impacts of lessening fiber consumption in individuals with persistent bowel obstruction — the direct inverse of what most specialists would suggest. Participants were told to consume no fiber at all for a long time. Then, at that point, they were permitted to build their fiber admission to a level they were OK with or follow a high-fiber diet.

Unbelievably, the majority of the subjects were doing great to such an extent that they picked to forge ahead with the zero-fiber plan. The review endured just half a year. The condition of those who consumed a lot of fiber did not change, but those who consumed little or no fiber saw significant improvements in their symptoms, including less gas, bloating, and straining. Moreover, the ones on zero fiber expanded the recurrence of their toilet usage - defecations!...

The school of thought that fiber-filled eating plans could be dangerous for the stomach isn't clear, however meat-only eating plan advocates fault specific mixtures in plant food varieties as the wellspring of stomach-related issues. They refer to the book The Plant Paradox, by Steven R. Gundry, M.D., which opines that the normal protection attributes that plants contain to deter pests result in bulging, gas, and other stomach-related trouble that might make them not worth eating for people. Lectins, gluten, and phytic corrosive — which are found normally in organic products, greens, beans, grains, nuts, and seeds — can add to irritation and auto-resistant problems like IBS, and that's only the tip of the iceberg. Although this is a point of contention, it does explain the claim that meat-only advocates feel better than when they eat plants.

6. Expanded Mental Lucidity

Similarly as with the ketogenic diet, advocates i.e. those who practice the meat-only eating plan report thinking all the more plainly and having better fixation practically immediately.

Once more, as with going keto, there is a break-in period where your body needs to sort out some way to fuel your framework without carbs, so you'll presumably feel dormant and grumpy from the start. You might experience issues resting and even foster awful breath (an early sign that your body is making ketones), yet you can brave it. Within a couple of days or a little more than seven days, you could feel more honed than at any other time. Maybe shockingly better than if you were doing a standard ketogenic diet.

7. Less Complex Eating Plan

There's one thing about the meat-only diet that nobody can contend with: it's not muddled up. You eat meat when you're ravenous, and that is all there is to it. If you're the sort of individual who gets confounded counting calories or macros, and is easily tired out on weighing segments on a food scale, or doesn't know what contains gluten and what doesn't, a meat-only eating plan will save you a lot of reasoning time. Also, keeping in mind that a meat-rich eating routine might seem like it would burn through every last cent, the sums you consume may not be high, since meat is so satisfying.

That ought to minimize expenses — particularly on the off chance that you in a real sense aren't going for some other food.

You probably now agree that the meat-only diet isn't quite as absurd as it seems at first. By and by, there are a few convincing motivations to not attempt it — or possibly not consider following it for an extended period — aside from what we've previously referenced, and on the flip side;

Here are the drawdowns of a meat-only eating plan;

1. Environmental Consequences

The impact on the environment If everyone followed this diet, the world would run out of animal sources pretty quickly. Supporting natural cultivating practices and eating locally is an honorable, savvy method for increasing the safety of animals and eradicating poisons, nevertheless, multiplying the need for meat would without a doubt negatively affect the planet — essentially while regular cultivating techniques stay prevalent.

2. Vegetables Are Still Great

Meat-only eating plan advocates fault stomach-related issues on plants. Grains, vegetables, and nuts are without a doubt wellsprings of antinutrients that can forestall the body's retention of iron and zinc. Although, plants have natural protection frameworks to deter pests and other harmful organisms from eating them, however, that doesn't mean they can't or ought not be eaten, just as other forms of life have their defensive structures, yet that doesn't suggest that you can't eat them too.

Likewise, how we process and prepare our food lessens the power of the antinutrients inside it. At the point when bread is prepared with yeast, the phytic corrosive substance in the grains disperses. Levels are likewise low in some types of grains and sourdough bread.

It is not necessarily the case that certain individuals aren't particularly delicate to specific plant food varieties. Assuming you know one that irritates you, don't eat it. However, it's most likely best not to get rid of all of the vegetation in your eating regimen because of the reaction of your body to a couple of types you've once eaten.

3. Supportability

The planet isn't the main thing that could be damaged assuming you go all meat, constantly. You might wind up detesting life, regardless of how cool eating burgers and bacon the entire day sounds to you now. Following an uncompromising meat-only eating plan implies no brew, no avocados for your Fajita Night… and, truth be told, no fajitas by any means (tortillas are a big NO!). You can twist the principles and have your cheat days, however, at that point you're not doing the eating regimen, or are you?

Conclusion

The meat-only eating plan enjoys numerous benefits, however, the logical and laboratory-affirmed information needs to keep up with the postulated benefits. Since the eating regimen is profoundly prohibitive and removes whole nutrition types, it may not be a suitable long-haul dietary plan for some people. Moreover, the harmlessness of the eating routine presently can't seem to be thoroughly affirmed. The eating regimen might expand the danger of cardiovascular infection and type 2 diabetes because of the eating routine's high consumption of meat and low consumption of plants. Talking with your physician about the expected dangers and advantages is a decent initial step before setting out on any eating routine arrangement, particularly one that is exceptionally prohibitive and removes whole nutrition classes.

Albeit a few recounted reports recommend that blockage of the bowels isn't an issue on a meat-only eating plan, even though you are avoiding fiber, which is a supplement significant for internal well-being.

Furthermore, an eating routine high in red and processed meats has been connected to a high rate of gastric cancer, and eating a lot of meat protein can likewise put excessive pressure on your kidneys. While this diet might sound insane to certain individuals I try to be as liberal as could be expected. Assuming there's a breakthrough eating plan that is working for individuals, I don't discredit that. But, all things considered, there is no investigation into the short- or long-term impacts of this particular eating routine, which makes it hazardous.

Likewise, with any eating routine, it's alright to explore different avenues regarding getting your nourishment, yet ensure it doesn't hurt you. Be reasonable about your well-being, and if your well-being is deteriorating and not improving, that is the ideal time to consider another arrangement because, in actual reality, no eating routine is a cure-all.

A little note from the author;

I'm sure you enjoyed reading this and gained some tips on how to live healthier. Kindly, do well to drop a review and visit my store on Amazon to check out some of my other writings;

https://www.amazon.com/author/williamwalker_writes

Thanks.